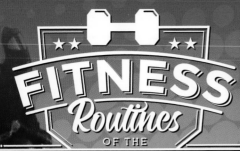

FITNESS
Routines
OF THE
SUPERSTAR ATHLETES

LINDSEY VONN

JEFF
SAVAGE

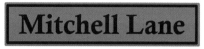

PUBLISHERS

2001 SW 31st Avenue
Hallandale, FL 33009

www.mitchelllane.com

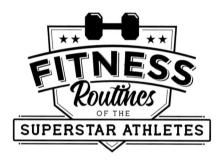

First Edition, 2020.
Author: Jeff Savage
Designer: Ed Morgan
Editor: Lisa Petrillo

Series: Fitness Routines of the Superstar Athletes
Title: Lindsey Vonn / by Jeff Savage

Hallandale, FL : Mitchell Lane Publishers, [2020]

Library bound ISBN: 9781680204711
eBook ISBN: 9781680204728

Contents

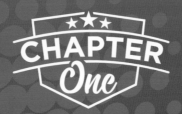

CHAPTER One

SPEED Racer

Lindsey Vonn stood in the start house and stared down the mountain. She was about to race in skiing's **downhill** event at the 2018 Olympic Games in Pyeongchang, South Korea. Vonn took deep breaths to calm herself and fidgeted with her pole straps. She knew what was at stake. She had already won more races than any female skier in history. Now she was trying to become the oldest woman ever to win an Olympic medal.

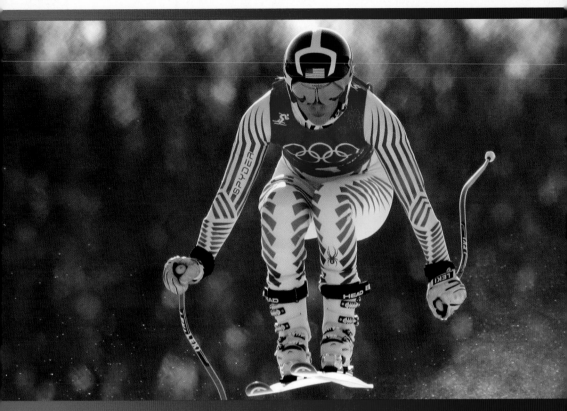

Vonn is determined to make history at the 2018 Olympic Games.

Vonn's family waited in the stands at the bottom of the course with thousands of other fans. "Every single meal she's eaten for the last two years is for this moment," said her sister Karin Kildow. "Every single gym workout. Every single thing she's done every day for the last eight years is for these next two minutes."

Vonn also understood the danger. Violent crashes had put her in the hospital more times than she cared to remember. Surgery scars marked her body. A metal rod ran through the length of her right arm. Her right knee had been rebuilt. But Vonn couldn't think about any of this now. Her focus was to ski as fast as possible.

5

Vonn bolted from the starting gate and went nearly straight down the slope. She shifted her weight from one foot to the other while keeping her skis together, digging their edges into the hard pack of the snow. Her slight turns formed the shape of skinny letter S's. Vonn was a master of the downhill. Eight years earlier at the Vancouver Olympics she had become the only American to win this race. She was favored to win the gold medal again at the 2014 Games but injuries kept her from competing. At age 33, she said this was her last chance. "In ski-racing age, I'm old," she said. "I want to keep racing forever, but my body can't take many more beatings."

Vonn needed a fearless performance. Two racers earlier, top-ranked Sofia Goggia of Italy had posted a blazing time of 1 minute, 39.22 seconds. Vonn tucked low and nearly flew down the hill. To safety officials alongside the course, she was a blur of red-white-and-blue, flashing by at 80 miles an hour. They certainly could not see the letters "DK" etched in her helmet. The initials stood for Don Kildow, Vonn's grandfather who taught her to ski. Kildow had served in the U.S. military during the Korean War 67 years earlier and hoped to return to the country to see his granddaughter compete in the Olympics. But he died three months earlier. Vonn was skiing for him.

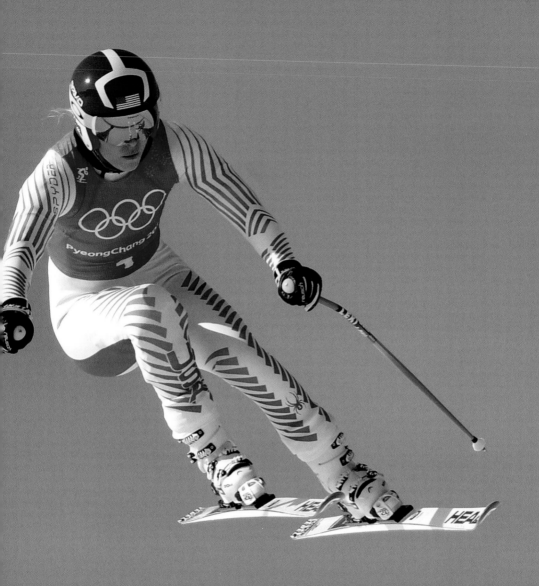

Vonn is fearless as she soars to new heights in
the dangerous Olympic downhill race.

Vonn dashed across the finish line and spun her head toward the timing scoreboard. It read: *1:39.69*. Second place. She smiled, waved to the cameras, and blew a kiss to the clouds for her grandfather. She didn't win gold but maybe she could still get a medal. The problem was, she was just the seventh racer to come down the course. There were still 32 racers to go. Soon enough, the 19th skier, Norway's Ragnhild Mowinckel, moved into second place for the silver medal. Vonn fell to third. All that was left was the bronze. Twenty racers remained. Across the line they came, one by one, as Vonn quietly fretted. When the final skier finished, Vonn smiled wide. She had won the bronze medal to become the oldest female ski medalist in Olympic history.

"I desperately wanted to win for my grandfather, but I still think he'd be proud of me," she told reporters as tears welled in her eyes. "I've been injured so many times and I worked really hard to get here. I won the bronze medal but I feel like I won the gold medal. I'm so thankful to be here. It's sad. It's my last downhill. I wish I could keep going."

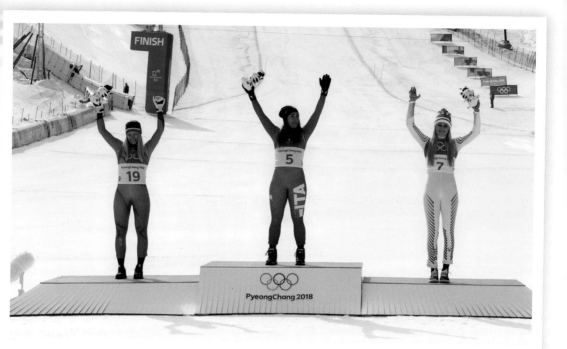

Vonn (*right*) is proud to represent the United States on the podium as she stands with the other 2018 Olympic downhill medalists Sofia Goggia of Italy (center) and Ragnhild Mowinckel of Norway.

Fun Fact

Lindsey's three dogs—Leo, Bear, and Lucy—have their own Instagram account as "Vonndogs."

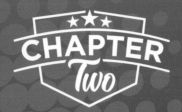

CHAPTER Two

TRAINING for Fame

Lindsey Caroline Kildow was born October 18, 1984, in Saint Paul, Minnesota. (She changed her last name to Vonn when she married.) Lindsey's parents, Alan and Linda, raised Lindsey in the nearby town of Burnsville along with her siblings Karin, Reed, Dylan, and Laura. Lindsey was 2 when her grandfather, Don Kildow, put her on skis for the first time. Lindsey's father competed in ski racing as a teen and trained under coach Erich Sailer.

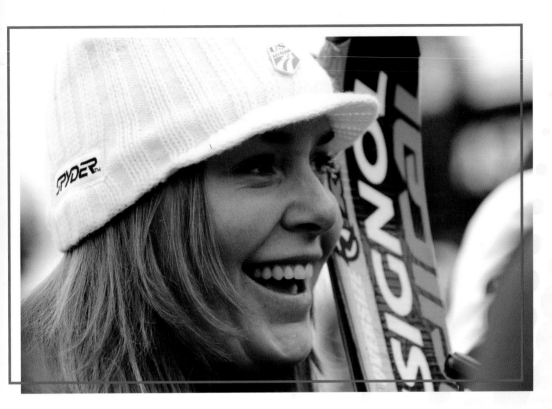

Lindsey's family supported her quest for glory.

When Lindsey was 6, her father took her to Buck Hill Ski Racing School where Sailer trained her. Lindsey improved quickly, and at age 7, she and her father made a five-year plan. Lindsey was 12 when her family left their home and moved to Vail, Colorado, so she could get year-round training. "I always dreamed I would be in the Olympics, but I was a kid, so it was kind of like a childish dream," Lindsey told a magazine writer. "Vail was wonderful to me, but I missed out on a normal childhood—sleepovers, school dances. And my brothers and sisters left their friends for me. I felt so guilty. It was a lot of pressure."

At Ski Club Vail, Lindsey joined the Gravity Corps youth club where she learned **all-mountain skills** and technical racing. She preferred keeping her skis in the **fall line** to go as fast as possible. To train in daylight, she was home-schooled so she could study at night. Her hard work paid off at age 14 when she became the first American female to win the Cadets **slalom** event at Trofeo Topolino in Italy. Famed U.S. skier Picabo Street, who was Lindsey's childhood hero, watched her compete in Italy.

"The faster she went, the bigger the smile she got on her face," Street told reporters. "You can't teach somebody to love the fall line like that little girl loved the fall line."

At age 17, Lindsey competed in the 2002 Olympic Games in Salt Lake City, Utah. She finished sixth in the **combined** and 32nd in the slalom. A year later she won her first World Cup medal (bronze). At the 2006 Torino Olympics in Italy, she finished seventh in the **super G** and eighth in the downhill. The following year she married Thomas Vonn, a skier who competed in the 2002 Olympics. In 2008, Lindsey won a U.S.-record 10 World Cup tour races and collected more points than any other racer to win the overall World Cup title.

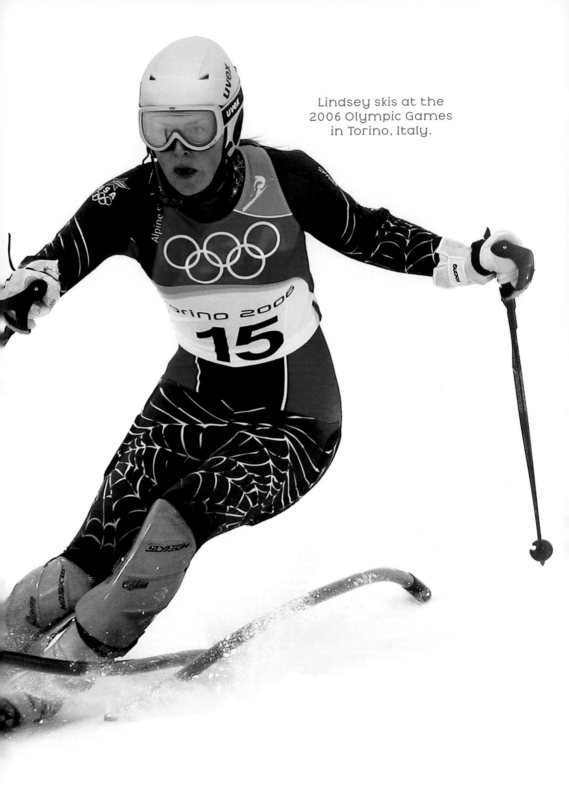

Lindsey skis at the 2006 Olympic Games in Torino, Italy.

She won the title again in 2009 and 2010 to break nearly every American record. In 2011, the Vonns announced their divorce.

Lindsey continued to reach even greater skiing wins. At age 26, she won the Olympic gold medal in Canada in the downhill. When she saw her name atop the leaderboard, she screamed for joy and fell to the snow. Three days later she won bronze in the super G. She was instantly famous.

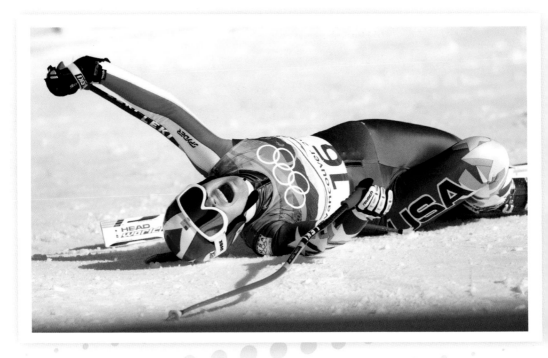

Vonn has reason to celebrate after becoming the first American to win the Olympic gold medal in the downhill at the 2010 Vancouver Games.

By 2012, she was nearly unbeatable as she claimed her fourth World Cup title. But the following year she suffered a serious knee injury that knocked her out of the 2014 Olympics. Vonn worked her way back. One year later she won her 63rd World Cup race, the most by any woman in world history. Only Sweden's Ingemar Stenmark, with his 86 victories, was in front of her now. Following the 2018 Olympics, Vonn planned to retire after one more World Cup season. She reached 82 wins and joked, "Not bad for an old lady." But then she suffered another knee injury. Her retirement plans changed. "I know I've said my body can't handle it anymore," she said. "But I'm thinking at this point that I need to come back."

Fun Fact

Vonn uses men's skis. At 5 feet 10 inches tall, she is larger than most women skiers. The longer men's skis require more strength to turn but provide more speed.

15

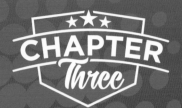

CHAPTER
Three

INTENSE
Fitness

It's no surprise that Vonn wants to keep racing. Injuries have never stopped her. At the 2006 Torino Olympics in Italy, she crashed during a practice run and had to be flown by helicopter to the hospital. She raced two days later. At the 2013 World Championships in Austria, she suffered torn knee ligaments and a broken leg. Doctors rebuilt her knee and said it would take one year for her to recover. Five months later she was skiing. She suffered a broken arm in a training crash in 2016, and two months later at an event in Germany she still couldn't move her arm well enough to put her hair in a ponytail. She insisted on racing anyway. She could not grip her ski pole, so she taped her glove to it. She won the race.

What makes Vonn unstoppable? It's her intense training program. Her rock-solid physique has prevented *more* injuries. When her high-speed risks do end with a bang, she recovers faster than others. As a teen, Lindsey exercised mostly by skiing. This changed after a bike ride with fellow skier Julia Mancuso in Lake Tahoe, California. Lindsey fell miles behind Mancuso. She was embarrassed and knew she needed to improve her training. She spent the next three summers in Monaco learning indoor training, moved her off-season training to Austria, and now has a personal trainer who travels the world with her. She spends more time in the gym than on the slopes. "She treats the training as part of her job," said her trainer, Alex Bunt. "She demands excellence. Everything we do is based on science."

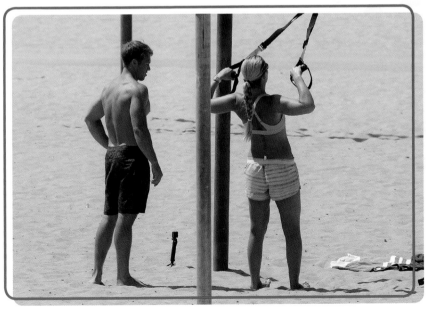

Alex Bunt trains with Vonn on TRX bands.

In the off-season, Vonn trains five days a week, five hours a day, at a Los Angeles gym. She starts a grueling morning session by gently exercising her rebuilt knee. She pedals a **stationary bike** to increase blood flow and heart rate. She continues warming up with an hour of stretching exercises. Next she does a series of **core** exercises, such as **twist tucks**, planks, and **anti-rotation holds**. An hour of strength work follows. This consists of lifting heavy weights, mainly for her lower body and core. She does **deadlifts**, **barbell squats**, and other power lifts. From there she performs **agility** exercises, such as **box jumps**, jumping rope, and jump squats as Bunt lightly pushes her during each jump to shift her landing spot. Next come exercises like forward and side **lunges**. The workout ends with balance exercises after her legs are tired. Vonn goes home for lunch and a recovery nap, then she returns to the gym for an intense stationary bike workout.

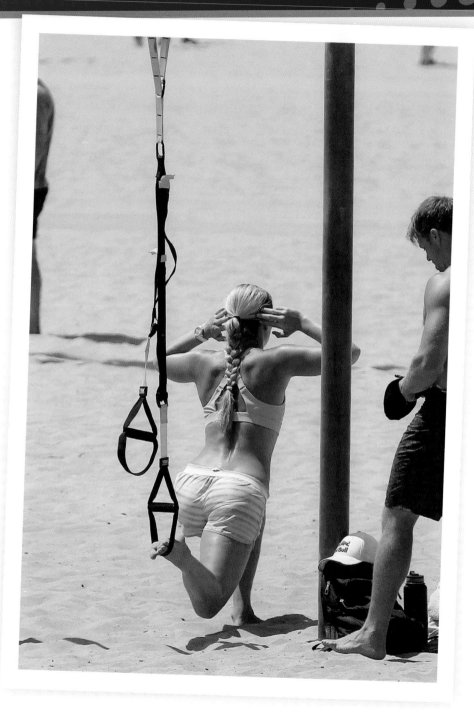

Vonn practices lunges with TRX bands
as Bunt instructs.

19

During the season, Vonn does two strength-training sessions each week and pedals the bike every day after skiing. "Her bike fitness is incredible," Bunt told a magazine writer. "She's a beast with her training. And she's super coachable. Tell her one thing and she fixes it. That's why she's so great." Vonn ices her knee for 20 minutes after every workout. She sleeps up to 10 hours each night. "I'm a big sleeper, that's how I recover," she said. "That way, I feel so much more energized and ready to go hard again the next day."

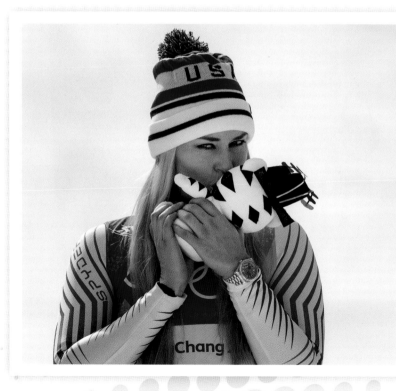

Vonn knows to work hard ... and sleep well.

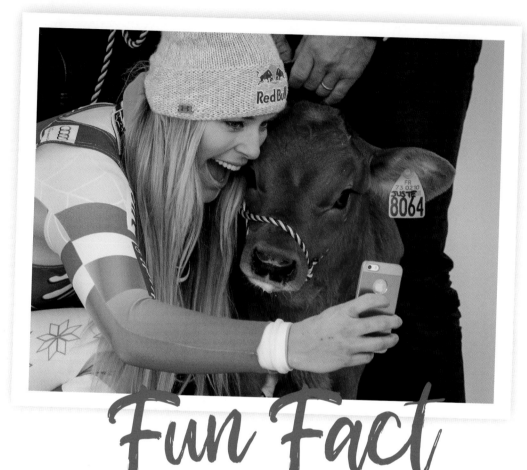

Fun Fact

After a race in Val d'Isere in 2014, Vonn was awarded a cow. She named her new pet Winnie. Vonn also won a calf in 2005, which has since had enough babies to give Vonn a small herd. Vonn keeps them on a farm in Austria.

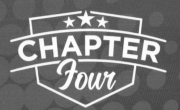

MINDFUL
Eating

Vonn is a planner. Her fitness routine is mapped out on a timeline for days, weeks, and months. She is just as aware of her nutrition. She knows her body needs certain amounts of carbohydrates for energy and protein for muscle development. She calls it "mindful eating." She has a personal chef who helps her with her meals. Her typical day might look like this:

Breakfast—scrambled eggs with red bell peppers, onions, mushrooms, avocado, and salsa, along with a bowl of oatmeal with cinnamon and blueberries.

Lunch—grilled chicken breast and a salad with walnuts, dried cranberries, and balsamic vinaigrette.

Dinner—spaghetti or other pasta with a piece of fish or chicken, green beans, and carrots.

Chapter FOUR

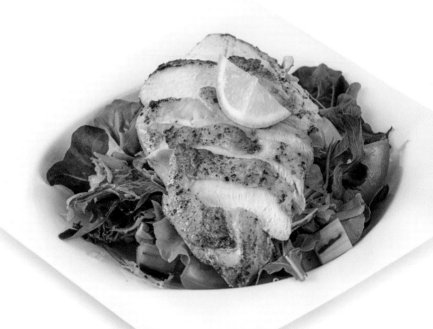

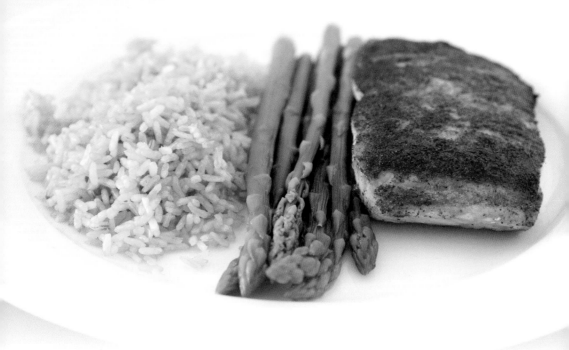

Vonn's favorite pre-race meal is salmon, asparagus, and brown or wild rice. To maintain her energy level through the day she eats snacks, such as protein shakes, oatmeal bars, or a handful of almonds. She also enjoys sweet potatoes, cauliflower mash, grain bowls, and colorful vegetables. She chooses the healthy option of similar foods: almond butter instead of peanut butter, pumpernickel bread instead of white bread, and her favorite secret trick—apple sauce instead of butter. She drinks 13 glasses of water a day.

Vonn's mindful eating might seem strict, but she understands the joy of eating. She makes exceptions, and she explains it this way: "I hate the word diet. You'll drive yourself insane if you only eat what you're supposed to eat. Everyone should have a treat once in a while. For me it might be frozen yogurt or banana bread. Or maybe even a Reese's Peanut Butter Cup or a bowl of Fruity Pebbles cereal. You want to eat smart and healthy. But you shouldn't stop eating things you really enjoy. Just try to be as active as you can."

Fun Fact

Lindsey tried other sports growing up, such as tennis and figure skating. "I was very bad at all of them," she said. "I was actually not so bad at gymnastics, but I was way too tall."

25

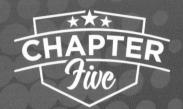

CHAPTER Five
LEADING the Way

Lindsey Vonn is the greatest American skier ever. She has won more races—by far—than any other woman in the world. Companies pay her millions of dollars to sponsor their products. She owns million-dollar homes in Colorado and California. But Vonn is not interested in being rich and famous. She prefers spending her time skiing, training, and helping others. Her charitable foundation features camps and **scholarships** for girls.

Vonn knows the importance of representing her sport, so she does photo shoots for magazine covers and appears on television talk shows. She even had fun acting in an episode of her favorite TV show—*Law & Order*. But she doesn't seek attention. "It's kind of awkward standing there while people take pictures of you," she told a magazine writer. "I definitely don't fit in on the red carpet. I'm like twice the size of the other women, in both height and weight. But that's even more of a reason to show girls that you don't have to be a certain size. Any size is beautiful. It's about being confident with who you are. I want girls to lead a healthy lifestyle and be happy."

Vonn recently wrote a book featuring tips on fitness and nutrition. In 2018, she joined with basketball superstar LeBron James, super model Cindy Crawford, and actor and former governor Arnold Schwarzenegger to form a health and wellness company. And despite her "old" age, as she calls it, she will keep ski racing as long as she can. "I've crashed into fences so many times and had so many injuries," she said. "I know so many doctors, it's ridiculous. But I'm also not a quitter. No matter what obstacle I face, I feel like I can overcome it. Who knows? Maybe there will be some medical miracle to fix my knee, and I'll be like Robo knee, and I'll ski for ten more years."

AWARDS

Sportswoman of the Year (U.S. Olympic Committee)
2 times (2009, 2010)

Female Athlete of the Year (Associated Press)
2010

World Skier of the Year
8 times (2003, 2004, 2006, 2007, 2008, 2009, 2012, 2016)

Olympic Medalist
3 times (2010, 2018)

Olympic Gold Medalist
(2010)

World Cup overall title
4 times (2008, 2009, 2010, 2012)

World Cup downhill title
8 times (2008-2013, 2015, 2016)

World Cup super G title
5 times (2009, 2010, 2011, 2012, 2015)

World Cup combined title
3 times (2010, 2011, 2012)

TIMELINE

1985 — born in Saint Paul, Minnesota

1987 — began skiing

1990 — started ski lessons

1997 — moved to Vail, Colorado

1999 — won the Cadets slalom in Italy

2002 — competed in the Salt Lake City Olympics

2006 — competed in the Torino Olympics

2007 — married Thomas Vonn

2008 — won first of three straight overall World Cup titles

2010 — won gold and bronze medals in the Vancouver Olympics

2012 — won fourth overall World Cup title

2013 — suffered major knee injury

2018 — won bronze medal in the Pyeongchang Olympics

GLOSSARY

agility The ability to move quickly and easily

all-mountain skills The ability to ski on different types of terrain and snow conditions

anti-rotation hold Exercise that improves stability and core strength in which you hold a handle attached to a cable at a certain angle and prevent your body from turning

barbell squat Exercise starting from a standing position in which you carefully place a barbell across your upper back and squat down as if sitting in a chair and stand back up

box jump Exercise starting from a standing position in which you squat and jump up and forward and land on a box in front of you

combined Ski racing event that combines the times of a downhill and slalom run

core Trunk or midsection of the body

deadlift Exercise starting from a standing position in which you bend down from your hips while keeping your back straight to grip a weighted barbell and return to a standing position

downhill Fastest of the ski racing events with narrow turns

fall line The fastest line from the skier directly down the mountain

lunge Exercise starting from a standing position in which you step with one leg in a certain direction and squat before pushing with that leg back to a standing position

scholarship Money and other aid given to students to help pay to attend school

slalom Ski racing event that involves skiing inside and around gate poles

stationary bike   A fitness device similar to a bicycle that does not move and is used to exercise legs and core

super G   Ski racing event that features speed similar to the downhill but with wider turns—also called super giant slalom

twist tuck   Exercise from a pushup position in which you place your legs on a large, rubber-like ball and pull it toward you as you twist to one side

FURTHER READING

Braun, Eric. *Lindsey Vonn*. Minneapolis, MN: Lerner Publications, 2017.

Dann, Sarah. *Lindsey Vonn*. New York: Crabtree Publishing Company, 2013.

Nagelhout, Ryan. *Lindsey Vonn.* New York: Gareth Stevens Publishing, 2016.

ON THE INTERNET

www.LindseyVonn.com
Vonn's official site

www.usskiandsnowboard.org
The U.S. ski team official site

www.olympic.org/alpine-skiing
The Olympic Games skiing official site

INDEX

ABOUT the AUTHOR

Jeff Savage is the award-winning author of more than 200 books for young readers. A former sportswriter for the *San Diego Union-Tribune*, Jeff's books have been read by millions. Jeff lives with his wife, Nancy, sons Taylor and Bailey, and dogs Tunes, Coach, Ace, Champ, Tank, and Lexi (that's six!) in Folsom, California. Jeff competed in one ski race and lost—to his girlfriend. So he married her.